# VACCINES:

# DO THEY WORK & DO THEY CAUSE AUTISM?

## A GUIDE FOR THOSE WHO WANT TO KNOW THE TRUTH ABOUT VACCINES

### DRR. JOHAN DOUSTEPH (PH)[1]

---

[1] See About the Author section

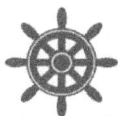

POINTS OF SAIL
PUBLISHING

Points of Sail Publishing
P.O. Box 30083 Prospect Plaza
FREDERICTON, New Brunswick
E3B 0H8, Canada

This book is not intended as a substitute for the medical advice of physicians. The reader should regularly consult a physician in matters relating to his/her health and particularly with respect to any symptoms that may require diagnosis or medical attention.

This book is sold with the understanding that the author and publisher are not providing any medical or professional advice. Though it provides its information in absolute terms, the author and publisher are neither for or against vaccines. This book is a parody, all names are fictitious, and you should consult your doctor for information regarding vaccines.

# ACKNOWLEDGEMENTS

The work of this book could not have been done without the countless many who've lost their lives. This book is for them.

Thank you all.

# 1. DO VACCINES WORK?

A Guide For Those Who Want to Know the Truth

YES, VACCINES WORK.

# A Guide For Those Who Want to Know the Truth

# 2. DO VACCINES CAUSE AUTISM?

NO, VACCINES DON'T CAUSE AUTISM.

# 3. WHAT CAN YOU DO WITH THIS INFORMATION TO HELP YOUR FAMILY?

STOP GOOGLING STUFF AND
GO TALK TO A DOCTOR.

A Guide For Those Who Want to Know the Truth

# Vaccines: Do They Work & Do They Cause Autism?

A Guide For Those Who Want to Know the Truth

# Vaccines: Do They Work & Do They Cause Autism?

# Vaccines: Do They Work & Do They Cause Autism?

# Vaccines: Do They Work & Do They Cause Autism?

.

# Vaccines: Do They Work & Do They Cause Autism?

# Vaccines: Do They Work & Do They Cause Autism?

# Vaccines: Do They Work & Do They Cause Autism?

# Vaccines: Do They Work & Do They Cause Autism?

# Vaccines: Do They Work & Do They Cause Autism?

# Vaccines: Do They Work & Do They Cause Autism?

# A Guide For Those Who Want to Know the Truth

# Vaccines: Do They Work & Do They Cause Autism?

# Vaccines: Do They Work & Do They Cause Autism?

A Guide For Those Who Want to Know the Truth

# Vaccines: Do They Work & Do They Cause Autism?

# Vaccines: Do They Work & Do They Cause Autism?

# Vaccines: Do They Work & Do They Cause Autism?

A Guide For Those Who Want to Know the Truth

# Vaccines: Do They Work & Do They Cause Autism?

# Vaccines: Do They Work & Do They Cause Autism?

# Vaccines: Do They Work & Do They Cause Autism?

A Guide For Those Who Want to Know the Truth

# Vaccines: Do They Work & Do They Cause Autism?

# A Guide For Those Who Want to Know the Truth

# Vaccines: Do They Work & Do They Cause Autism?

# Vaccines: Do They Work & Do They Cause Autism?

A Guide For Those Who Want to Know the Truth

# Vaccines: Do They Work & Do They Cause Autism?

# A Guide For Those Who Want to Know the Truth

# Vaccines: Do They Work & Do They Cause Autism?

# Vaccines: Do They Work & Do They Cause Autism?

# Vaccines: Do They Work & Do They Cause Autism?

# Vaccines: Do They Work & Do They Cause Autism?

# Vaccines: Do They Work & Do They Cause Autism?

# Vaccines: Do They Work & Do They Cause Autism?

# A Guide For Those Who Want to Know the Truth

# Vaccines: Do They Work & Do They Cause Autism?

# Vaccines: Do They Work & Do They Cause Autism?

# Vaccines: Do They Work & Do They Cause Autism?

# Vaccines: Do They Work & Do They Cause Autism?

# Vaccines: Do They Work & Do They Cause Autism?

# Vaccines: Do They Work & Do They Cause Autism?

# A Guide For Those Who Want to Know the Truth

# Vaccines: Do They Work & Do They Cause Autism?

# Vaccines: Do They Work & Do They Cause Autism?

# Vaccines: Do They Work & Do They Cause Autism?

# Vaccines: Do They Work & Do They Cause Autism?

Vaccines: Do They Work & Do They Cause Autism?

# Vaccines: Do They Work & Do They Cause Autism?

# Vaccines: Do They Work & Do They Cause Autism?

# Vaccines: Do They Work & Do They Cause Autism?

# Vaccines: Do They Work & Do They Cause Autism?

# Vaccines: Do They Work & Do They Cause Autism?

# Vaccines: Do They Work & Do They Cause Autism?

A Guide For Those Who Want to Know the Truth

# Vaccines: Do They Work & Do They Cause Autism?

# Vaccines: Do They Work & Do They Cause Autism?

# Vaccines: Do They Work & Do They Cause Autism?

# Vaccines: Do They Work & Do They Cause Autism?

# Vaccines: Do They Work & Do They Cause Autism?

A Guide For Those Who Want to Know the Truth

# Vaccines: Do They Work & Do They Cause Autism?

# Vaccines: Do They Work & Do They Cause Autism?

# Vaccines: Do They Work & Do They Cause Autism?

# Vaccines: Do They Work & Do They Cause Autism?

# Vaccines: Do They Work & Do They Cause Autism?

# Vaccines: Do They Work & Do They Cause Autism?

# Vaccines: Do They Work & Do They Cause Autism?

# Vaccines: Do They Work & Do They Cause Autism?

# Vaccines: Do They Work & Do They Cause Autism?

# Vaccines: Do They Work & Do They Cause Autism?

# Vaccines: Do They Work & Do They Cause Autism?

# A Guide For Those Who Want to Know the Truth

# Vaccines: Do They Work & Do They Cause Autism?

# Vaccines: Do They Work & Do They Cause Autism?

# Vaccines: Do They Work & Do They Cause Autism?

# Vaccines: Do They Work & Do They Cause Autism?

# Vaccines: Do They Work & Do They Cause Autism?

# Vaccines: Do They Work & Do They Cause Autism?

# Vaccines: Do They Work & Do They Cause Autism?

# Vaccines: Do They Work & Do They Cause Autism?

# Vaccines: Do They Work & Do They Cause Autism?

# Vaccines: Do They Work & Do They Cause Autism?

# Vaccines: Do They Work & Do They Cause Autism?

# Vaccines: Do They Work & Do They Cause Autism?

A Guide For Those Who Want to Know the Truth

# Vaccines: Do They Work & Do They Cause Autism?

# Vaccines: Do They Work & Do They Cause Autism?

# Vaccines: Do They Work & Do They Cause Autism?

# Vaccines: Do They Work & Do They Cause Autism?

# Vaccines: Do They Work & Do They Cause Autism?

# Vaccines: Do They Work & Do They Cause Autism?

# Vaccines: Do They Work & Do They Cause Autism?

# Vaccines: Do They Work & Do They Cause Autism?

# Vaccines: Do They Work & Do They Cause Autism?

# Vaccines: Do They Work & Do They Cause Autism?

# Vaccines: Do They Work & Do They Cause Autism?

# Vaccines: Do They Work & Do They Cause Autism?

# Vaccines: Do They Work & Do They Cause Autism?

# Vaccines: Do They Work & Do They Cause Autism?

# Vaccines: Do They Work & Do They Cause Autism?

# Vaccines: Do They Work & Do They Cause Autism?

# Vaccines: Do They Work & Do They Cause Autism?

# Vaccines: Do They Work & Do They Cause Autism?

# Vaccines: Do They Work & Do They Cause Autism?

# Vaccines: Do They Work & Do They Cause Autism?

# Vaccines: Do They Work & Do They Cause Autism?

# Vaccines: Do They Work & Do They Cause Autism?

# Vaccines: Do They Work & Do They Cause Autism?

# Vaccines: Do They Work & Do They Cause Autism?

# Vaccines: Do They Work & Do They Cause Autism?

# Vaccines: Do They Work & Do They Cause Autism?

# Vaccines: Do They Work & Do They Cause Autism?

# Vaccines: Do They Work & Do They Cause Autism?

# Vaccines: Do They Work & Do They Cause Autism?

# Vaccines: Do They Work & Do They Cause Autism?

# Vaccines: Do They Work & Do They Cause Autism?

# Vaccines: Do They Work & Do They Cause Autism?

# Vaccines: Do They Work & Do They Cause Autism?

# Vaccines: Do They Work & Do They Cause Autism?

# Vaccines: Do They Work & Do They Cause Autism?

# Vaccines: Do They Work & Do They Cause Autism?

A Guide For Those Who Want to Know the Truth

# Vaccines: Do They Work & Do They Cause Autism?

# Vaccines: Do They Work & Do They Cause Autism?

# THE END

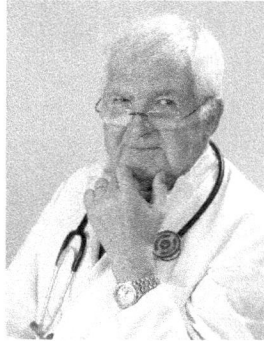

# ABOUT THE AUTHOR

DRR. Johan Dousteph (PH) is not a real person, not a doctor, has no PhD. and as such makes no claims to any medical knowledge.

The picture you see above is a stock photo, and all quotes are fictional and all names made up.

You should talk to a real doctor about vaccines. There are countless studies proving that vaccines work, and that they don't cause autism. Your physician is the best one to provide you with any and references as they should be the one you get your advice from.

This book is not intended as a substitute for the medical advice of physicians. The reader should regularly consult a physician in matters relating to his/her health and particularly with respect to any symptoms that may require diagnosis or medical attention.

www.ingramcontent.com/pod-product-compliance
Lightning Source LLC
Chambersburg PA
CBHW050503210326
41521CB00011B/2302